Clinical Pharmacy: A Practical Manual

www.lulu.com
Lulu Press, Inc
627 Davis Drive, Suite 300,
Morrisville, NC 27560.

Affiliation of Authors

Dr. Sagar Pamu	**Dr. Parameshwar Ravula**
Associate Professor,	Professor,
Pharmacy Practice Department,	Department of Pharmaceutical Chemistry,
Amity Institute of Pharmacy,	Amity Institute of Pharmacy,
Amity University,	Amity University,
Gwalior, Madhya Pradesh, India, 474005.	Gwalior, Madhya Pradesh, India, 474005.

First Printing: 2023
ISBN: 9781312672604
Copyright License @ Sagar Pamu

All rights reserved. This book or any portion thereof may not be reproduced or used in any manner whatsoever without the express written permission of the publisher except for the use of brief quotations in a book review or scholarly journal.

Clinical Pharmacy: A Practical Manual

Author

Sagar Pamu
Parameshwar Ravula

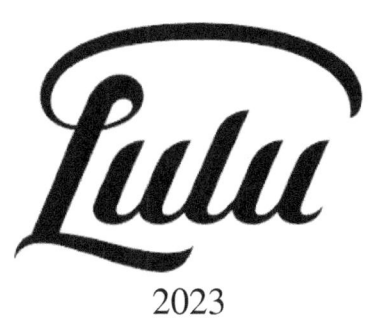

2023

About the Author

Dr. Sagar Pamu, Associate Professor of Amity Institute of Pharmacy, Amity University, Gwalior, Madhya Pradesh, India. He authored 24 books and published 24 research and case report papers in national and international journals. He also filed one patent. He participated and given many poster and oral presentations in various national and international conferences, workshops, or symposiums. He is a reviewer in 3 reputed journals indexed with scopus and web of science. He achieved a Young Scientist Award.

Dr. Parameshwar Ravula is a Professor of Amity Institute of Pharmacy, Amity University, Madhya Pradesh obtained his Ph.D. in Pharmaceutical Sciences from Jawaharlal Nehru Technological University, Hyderabad, India. He has contributed 30 papers in various SCI and Scopus indexed National & International Journals. He has 15 years of teaching experience in the field of pharmacy. He is also a member of several professional bodies.

Acknowledgments

At the very outset, I thank God, the Almighty for showering his blessings and being a source of guidance and wisdom throughout the study without which no human achievement is possible.

I indebted to our beloved **Parents** without whose encouragement and help our professional career would never see the light of the day.

As we walk along the path of life, I have a pleasure of meeting people who search our life in such a way that it never is the same gain…it may be small thoughtful things they do, a smile, a helping hand, a word of encouragement or just by mere presence they make our life worth living.

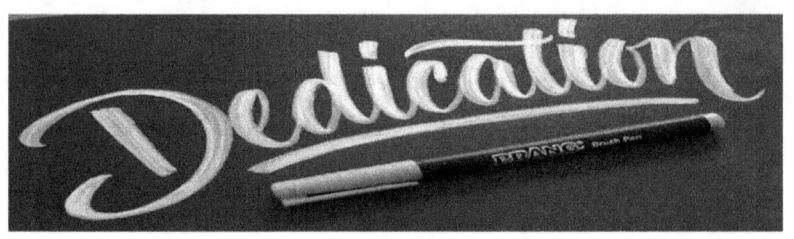

We thank our God Sri Venkateshwara Swamy for his gracious blessings.

Table of Contents

ANSWERING DRUG INFORMATION QUERIES 1

PATIENT MEDICATION COUNSELLING 16

INTERPRETATIONS OF LABORATORY INVESTIGATIONS 28

PATIENT MEDICATION HISTORY INTERVIEW 47

ADVERSE DRUG REACTION DETECTION & MANAGEMENT ... 58

MEDICATION ERRORS 76

DRUG UTILIZATION EVALUATION 83

Experiment No: 1

ANSWERING DRUG INFORMATION QUERIES

AIM: To discuss a brief introduction on answering drug information questions

INTRODUCTION:

Drug information is characterized by its function in responding orally or in writing to inquiries from a variety of healthcare professionals, patients, organizations, panels, and the general public regarding drug treatment and medications.

Drug information services can be applied to any activity where information about drug use is transmitted, including patient-related parts of pharmacy treatment. Drug information services' main activity is to provide precise and comprehensive information about drug use to pharmacies.

Pharmacists (or other healthcare experts) specializing in informing the public or other professionals about medications run drug information centers.

The drug information center offers trustworthy, impartial information to medical personnel, gives people individualized counselling and health information, and tracks and records inadequate drug responses.

Clinical pharmacy has a specialization called drug information. A chemist who specializes in medication information has the expertise and tools needed to utilize the information at their disposal.

A drug information service combines a variety of information sources, and the expertise of a professional chemist makes the service more useful than the sum of its parts.

Only if we center our practice on all available data and apply this information to patient treatment can the worth of medication therapy be maximized.

The Pharmacists and doctors drug information center (DIC) offers an impartial, comprehensive source of crucial medication knowledge to satisfy the requirements of working healthcare professionals. The different sources of knowledge about drugs can be divided into primary, secondary, and tertiary resources.

Primary resources:

Primary literature describes singular experiences that alter the world in terms of the knowledge that is currently accessible. They serve as the cornerstone upon which all other drug-related knowledge is built. These include journal articles on drug-related topics, such as case studies, pharmacological research, and accounts of clinical drug trials.

Medical and therapeutics Journal:

- British Medical Journal.
- Journal of the medical association.
- New England Journal of Medicine.

Pharmacy journals:

- American Journal of Hospital Pharmacy.
- Clinical Pharmacy.
- DICP-Annals of pharmacotherapy.
- Journal of Clinical and Hospital Pharmacy.

Drug and Toxicology Information and Pharmacology Journal.

- British Journal of Clinical Pharmacology.
- Human and Experimental Toxicology.

Secondary sources:

Review articles of original reports make up secondary sources. These offer a unique viewpoint on the literature and may also contain suggestions for practical applications of the theory.

- Medline
- IOWA Drug Information Service
- DRUGDEX
- Martindale
- POISINDEX

Tertiary resources:

Summaries of primary and secondary published literature make up tertiary resources. The primary example is printed textbooks, which are distinguished by a slow rate of revision in comparison to supplementary sources.

- AHFS-Drug Information Book
- Australian Medicine Handbook
- Basic skills in interpreting Lab data
- Drug information handbook
- Drug interactions Stockley
- Handbook of injectable
- Harrisons Principles of Internal Medicine
- Martindale
- Pharmacopoeias,
- BNF
- USP
- Australian formulary

AIMS AND OBJECTIVES OF DRUG INFORMATION SERVICES (DIC):

1. To satisfy the demands of medical professionals by offering an ordered catalogue source of knowledge on specialty drugs.
2. To offer impartial medical knowledge to nurses, doctors, and other health care workers in the hospital and community sectors.
3. To assist local healthcare experts by responding to their questions about different drugs.
4. To acknowledge and instruct on the value of assessment and to keep an eye on the accuracy of medication information.
5. To prepare recent pharmaceutical grads to act as knowledgeable sources of medical information.
6. Outline the fundamental conditions for creating DIC at different stages.
7. To offer a learning facility about medication knowledge skills to staff, student pharmacists, and other health sciences students.
8. To promote clinical pharmacist healthcare services by providing medication information services across the province.
9. To advertise the pharmacist vocation in different areas of medicine.
10. To provide evidence-based treatment by fostering patient care through the prudent use of medications.

FUNCTIONS OF DIC:

1. It gives information to healthcare workers and helps to refresh their understanding of medication information when there is not enough time for thorough study.
2. Sustain and create tradition based on pharmacoeconomics, institution-specific variables, and empirical proof of efficacy and wellbeing.
3. DIC organizes and promotes numerous initiatives on population-based drug practices to better patient results.
   Examples include creating standards for pharmacotherapy, therapeutic use criteria, and therapeutic exchange procedures.

4. Creates numerous initiatives to prevent prescription mistakes and adverse drug effects, such as monitoring, assuring institutional conformance with risk assessment and reduction strategies, and overseeing reporting and analysis programs (e.g., Med Watch).
5. The Food and Drug Administration (FDA), drug makers, and other sources watch and evaluate the distributed prescription safety warnings.
6. A variety of medical workers, patients, and caretakers receive drug information. By assessing procedures and participating in institutional review board committees, it also expanded its services in coordinating research services.
7. Create procedures for the restricted use of medicines and identify and handle substitute therapies for different illnesses based on formularies.
8. Constantly contributes to the provision of services for health care workers' schooling.
9. Takes part in high-calibre medication expense studies and development research initiatives.
10. Participates in peer evaluation of different scientific, literary, and study works.

BENEFITS OF DRUG INFORMATION SERVICES

- ❖ Encourages the safe and efficient use of medications by highlighting any medication-related issues in the order.
- ❖ Encouraging excellent professional care practices reduces the likelihood of drug-related problems for patients, significantly reducing the impact of drug misuse on society

.

- ❖ It offers medication-use rules and contributes to their processing in the creation of resources, passing this knowledge to different healthcare experts.
- ❖ By raising the pharmacy's efficiency, the amount of time healthcare professionals must spend examining medication knowledge is reduced.

Answering Drug Information Queries

- ❖ Enhance patient safety and obedience, which eventually promotes drug retention.
- ❖ Drug information services improve drug cost management by decreasing prescription misuse and raising patient and practitioner happiness.

PROCEDURE:

Step 1: Requester's details:

- Recognize the inquirer and get enough contact information.
- This information for recurring customers should be stored in a database to make future inquiries easier.
- Determine the level of reaction necessary.
- While less experienced employees may also seek advice on clinical administration, experienced doctors will likely favour succinct accurate information.
- There should always be an agreed-upon timeframe for an answer.
- Regarding professional queries, this frequently pertains to patient mobility requirements, treatment schedules, and staff schedules.
- An anticipated reaction time should be given if a specified date is not.
- The enquirer can be informed, and a new date can be discussed if this needs to be prolonged to handle the problem correctly.

Step 2: Background information:

- The inquirer can obtain more information, but it should be specific to the issue at hand and avoid attempting to cover all relevant clinical information.
- It is a challenging stage that requires clinical pharmacist expertise to get the most out of this early information sharing.
- Additional details, such as age, other medical conditions, kidney and hepatic function, other pertinent medications (including conventional drugs), a history of adverse responses, and the stage of pregnancy, may need to be gathered.

Step 3: Refine and categorize the question:

- After accepting the query, it might be essential to comprehend some of its components before looking for a response.
- For pharmacists, this is relevant, particularly to medical jargon and facets of illness and disease.
- Using this data clarifies the query and determines how long it will take to get a suitable answer.
- Because all inquiries must be completed within the limits of the available resources and the necessary timeline, this is crucial.
- There is a decreasing yield regarding improved quality or trust in the response after a certain point because it is uncommon to produce a flawless response.
- For therapeutic applications, a brief and prompt answer will be favoured over one that is detailed and time-consuming.
- Of course, for study endeavours, the opposite is true.
- The character of almost all medication information inquiries can be categorized, and this will determine the most effective and fruitful approach.

Step 4: Develop a strategy and search:

- Please take into account all of the information sources that are accessible and prioritize them based on the likelihood that the needed information will be found.
- There will frequently be no need to try a literature search because starting with primary sources (textbooks) and moving on to secondary literature will usually yield an acceptable response.
- In addition to using written and internet tools, consulting an expert or more seasoned coworker for advice might be feasible.
- It may also be required to use first principles; for instance, it may not be known how a medication will behave in renal failure. However, it can be anticipated based on its chemical and how renal replacement treatment is used (dialysis or hemofiltration).

- Keep track of the tools used and an overview of the information obtained. However, only the most pertinent references must be listed in the response.

Step 5: Interpret data:

- The information obtained needs to be thoroughly analyzed in light of the inquiry.
- It is crucial to consider the uniformity of information across different sources and whether clinical study applies to your community or a particular case.
- Whenever feasible, the complete text of reports that have been published should be reviewed because it is frequently the specifics—such as how patients were chosen for an experiment, how the medication was administered, and study limitations—that will aid in the analysis of particular questions.
- Pure solutions are uncommon in medication knowledge, so you might be the individual someone turns to in the last instance for an explanation.
- It is necessary to summarize and include this absence of confidence in an answer because there are frequently gaps in the data and contradictory studies or views.
- Nevertheless, professional judgments must still be made, and you might be asked to provide patient care recommendations in a setting with scant proof.

Step 6: Formulate and respond:

- The enquirer should receive a formed response as soon as possible, and answers should only be derived after closely analyzing the information found through a thorough search. All answers should be recorded in as much detail as required to support the statement.
- Even vocal answers given in a hurry should include the sources consulted and the query and answer.

- It should be repeated to ensure that the query has been understood correctly.
- Doctors prefer clear, succinct responses, but this does not negate the need to document and reference all pertinent information within the medication information service.
- When answering, additional (and occasionally foreseeable), inquiries frequently arise; offering more information is helpful if this happens.
- If a written statement is offered, say the reaction first, then provide specifics to support it. Write a report that does not conclude with a well-reasoned thesis.
- Every written answer should follow a formula that contains the query and your service's contact information (as you have interpreted it).
- Before making contact, if you are replying by phone, write down the key points you must make.
- A comprehensive log can be finished later for critical replies, but it is easy to get sidetracked during phone calls, so you must be careful to cover all your key points.
- State the question again at the start of the discussion so that the person asking it can concentrate on it and ensure you understand it correctly.

Step 7: Follow-up and document the outcome:

- Make an effort to ascertain the effects of your recommendations and any patient results.
- Although only feasible in a hospital or clinic, this is essential to learning how to provide drug information.
- The advice given should be documented in at least one form of paperwork (logbook, paper worksheet, computer programme).
- Drug information pharmacists have many skills and information tools at their disposal, but they frequently lack input and the chance to gain knowledge from practical practice.

- Clinical pharmacists who are currently in practice have the benefit of receiving ongoing instruction based on how their patients respond to treatments.
- Patient care areas with drug information services are more likely to get this crucial input from customers and coworkers.
- Input can also be requested by phone, email, or written inquiry.
- Whenever feasible, add results to the inquiry document.
- This data can be obtained to aid in upcoming replies if query records are stored.

Study questions:

1. Define drug information bulletin.
2. What is the role of the pharmacist in drug information service?
3. Explain the role of DIC and its relationship with various healthcare professionals.
4. Discuss the requirement of Drug and poison Information centers.
5. Explain the systematic approach in answering the drug information query.
6. Differences between DIC and PIC.
7. Critical Evaluation of Drug Information Literature.
8. Preparation of written and verbal drug information query reports and documentation.
9. List out the skills required for drug information specialists.

Answering Drug Information Queries

DRUG INFORMATION REQUEST AND DOCUMENTATION FORM

DI Code No:

Received date: **Received time:**

Received By:

Name of Enquirer:

Designation: **Phone No:**
Unit:

Professional status:

☐ Physician   ☐ Surgeon   ☐ Resident   ☐ Interns

☐ Pharmacist   ☐ Nurse   ☐ Others _____

☐ PG's (specify) _____

Query:

Information

Mode of request:

☐ Direct Access   ☐ During Ward Rounds   ☐ Telephone

☐ Email   ☐ Others

Purpose of enquiry:

☐ Updated Knowledge   ☐ Better Patient Care (if yes give details below)

☐ Others

Answer Needed

☐ Immediately   ☐ Within 2-4 hrs.   ☐ Within 1-2 days

☐ Within a day	
Delay for an answer (if any)	
Question Category:	
☐ Drug therapy ☐ Pregnancy/Lactation ☐ Indications	
☐ Poisoning ☐ Efficacy ☐ Stability	
☐ Pharmacokinetics/Pharmacodynamics ☐ Identification	
☐ Dose/administration Incompatibility ☐	
Patient Details:	
Age: Weight: Sex: Allergies:	
Current Medical Problem:	
Hepatic/Renal function details:	
Pregnancy/ lactation: Y/N (If yes give details)	
Other important investigations:	
Drug therapy:	

Answering Drug Information Queries

Query response:

References:

Textbook (mention):

Journals (mention):

Lexicomp:

Independent Drug Information Service:

Website:

Others (specify):

Mode of reply:

☐ Written ☐ Verbal ☐ Both

☐ Printed Literature ☐ Mail

Date of Reply: **Time of Reply:**

Follow up (if any):

Reporting Date:	**Reporting Time:**
Name of Pharmacists:	**Signature:**
Enquirer Department:	**Enquirer Email Id:**
Enquirer Sign:	

Experiment No: 2

PATIENT MEDICATION COUNSELLING

AIM: Introduction-Patient medication counselling

OBJECTIVES OF PATIENT COUNSELLING

1. The patient should understand how crucial his medicine is to his overall health.
2. It is essential to increase patient comprehension of how to cope with medical complications and adverse effects.
3. Must guarantee improved patient cooperation.
4. Creating a professional partnership and a framework for ongoing communication and collaboration is essential.
5. User takes an engaged, effective, and knowledgeable role in managing their health.
6. The chemist should be regarded as a specialist who provides pharmacological treatment.

INTRODUCTION:

1. Patient counselling is crucial to clinical pharmacy work in a hospital and community pharmacy environments.
2. Counselling helps people better comprehend their condition and how to manage it.
3. Check the patient's comprehension by providing comments.
4. Conclude by highlighting important aspects.
5. Allow the sufferer to voice any issues they may have.
6. Aid the sufferer in short follow-up.

DEFINITION:

Patient counselling gives patients knowledge, guidance, and support to use their medicines correctly. The chemist provides the patient or the patient's agent with information and guidance, which may also include suggestions for changing the patient's lifestyle or information about the patient's condition. Although it has typically spoken, the knowledge may also be provided in writing.

During counselling, the pharmacist should gauge the patient's comprehension of his or her condition and course of therapy and offer tailored guidance and information to help the patient take medicines most securely and efficiently as possible.

The pharmacy should know the etiology and treatments of the patient's illness to give correct guidance and information.

Gaining the patient's trust and inspiring them to follow the prescribed routine take practical communication skills.

COMMUNICATION SKILLS FOR EFFECTIVE COUNSELLING

Communication techniques, both **verbal** and **nonverbal**, are used in counselling. Language and paralinguistic elements like tone, loudness, intonation, and speaking pace are all part of verbal conversation. How we talk affects how patients understand a message because 40% of communication is paralinguistic or how we pronounce things.

- ❖ **Language:** Use straightforward English when conversing with patients and avoid superfluous medical jargon. Speak the patient's tongue if you can.
- ❖ **Tone:** During counselling, our vocal tone has a significant influence on the comprehension of the patient. Pitch range and level variations reveal the speaker's emotions and views. The speech should be comforting and compassionate when offering to counsel.
- ❖ **Volume:** Depending on the circumstance, the location, and the audience, many individuals talk at wildly varying volumes. Counselling should ideally take place in a calm, confidential situation where speaking aloud is not required. Most deaf patients profit more if the speaker steps closer and focuses their voice

towards the patient's ear, even though it may be required to talk more forcefully to patients with hearing impairments.

- ❖ **Speed:** Our speaking pace affects how clearly, we communicate. Because they may think the pharmacy is too preoccupied, patients may be hesitant to talk with a pharmacist who speaks rapidly. This might occur if the chemist is tense or unsure of the information provided. In comparison, someone who talks too slowly risks losing the listener's attention.

Non-verbal communication: This includes physical cues like the way the body, limbs, and head move and is positioned, as well as other things like how the pharmacy is clothed. Body language accounts for about 50% of the messages in any encounter. Nearness, touch, eye contact, facial emotions, head movements, hand and limb actions, and body positions are all examples of non-verbal communication.

Proximity: This refers to the separation that individuals keep during counselling. Four zones have been assigned to this area:

- ➢ Intimate (45 cm or less)
- ➢ Personal (45 cm to 1.2 m)
- ➢ Social (1.2–3.6 m)
- ➢ Public (>3.6 m)

Generally, counsellors and healthcare professionals use intimate or personal proximities.

- ❖ **Eye contact:** When discussing, people glance at each other more or less based on whether they are saying or hearing. Listeners focus on the speaker more frequently and for extended stretches of time. Some people might shy away from staring the therapist in the eyes due to societal or psychological factors like shyness, sorrow, or despair.
- ❖ **Facial expression:** Face expressions can show concern for the sufferer during counselling. Head motions like nodding, hand gestures, and body stances are also helpful.

PROCEDURE:

Steps of Patient Counselling

Since there are two distinct dialogue processes involved, the connection between the patient and the doctor is essential for the effectiveness of counselling.

Preparing for the session:

- The counsellor's expertise and knowledge are essential to the effectiveness of counselling.
- The chemist should be as knowledgeable as feasible about the patient and the specifics of his or her therapy. This can be done in a medical environment by consulting the patient's case records.
- In a neighbourhood drugstore, the patient, their prescription, and occasionally a log of the patient's prior dispensing are sources of information.
- A drug information source should be contacted before counselling begins if the chemist is inexperienced with the patient's medicine.
- The patient's bodily and emotional health should also be taken into account.
- Effective patient counselling is challenging if the patient is hurried, in discomfort, or non-communicative.
- In such cases, counselling goals might need to be changed, or the appointment might be postponed with the patient's consent.

Opening the session:

- Information collecting occurs during the first stage of counselling.
- The pharmacist should announce themselves and address the customer by name.
- If you need assistance saying the patient's name, approach a coworker or the person directly.
- It is preferable to start with an honorific like Ms, Mrs, or Mr and then use the first name.

Patient Medication Counselling

- The chemist needs to make it very obvious what the session's goals are.

Counselling content: The counselling material is regarded as the focal point of the counselling discussion. The chemist talks to the patient about his or her medicines and therapy plan at this stage. Changing one's lifestyle through food or fitness may also be addressed.

Topics commonly covered include:

- The drug's brand and dosage information.
- The rationale behind the prescription (if known) or how it functions.
- Medication dosage instructions (how much and how often).
- The anticipated length of therapy.
- The anticipated advantages of therapy.
- Potential adverse effects.
- Potential drug or food conflicts.
- Suggestions for proper storing.
- A minimal time frame is needed to demonstrate the treatment effect.
- What to do in case of skipped dosage.
- Particular surveillance needs, such as blood work.

Closing the session:

- Confirming that the patient has understood before the lesson ends are crucial.
- Feedback inquiries like, "Can you recall what this medicine is for?" can be used to evaluate this. Alternatively, "How long do you need to take this medication?"
- The patient may have met some of his or her knowledge requirements during the conversation, but there may still be unanswered concerns or uncertainties.

- Therefore, asking the patient if they have any concerns before ending the appointment is recommended.
- Before concluding, if time allows, briefly restate the key ideas in a rational sequence.
- If appropriate, the pharmacy can give their phone number to the patient in order to urge them to call if they require any additional guidance or information.

Getting Started

- For newcomers, patient counselling may seem intimidating. Students and recent graduates should have the chance to watch a seasoned chemist offer counselling to various patients.
- This gives the student or chemist the courage to get started and prepares them for encounters during a routine counselling appointment.
- A helpful strategy for freshly graduated pharmacists who lack trust in counselling is to begin by restricting counselling to a specific class of medication, such as oral hypoglycemia drugs.
- Who can be counselled in hospitals and neighbourhood shops frequently depends on staffing levels and available time.
- Due to the high patient volume, pharmacists may need to recognize and give precedence to those patients who need counselling the most.

These may include:

Patients taking specialized medications, such as antibiotics or medications with a limited therapeutic window, like warfarin, theophylline, or methotrexate;

Patients taking complicated medication regimes, like anti-tubercular medications Patients receiving medicines via specialized delivery methods, such as

- inhalers and rotohalers,

- patients with a history of noncompliance with medication regimens,
- elderly patients taking multiple medications, and
- patients are getting ready to leave the hospital, Individuals that doctors have recommended.

Counselling Aids

When information is given to a patient orally, there is a possibility that the patient may eventually lose the information. To help in patient counselling, numerous teaching and educational tools have been created. The patient can review the material at their ease as and when it is needed if it is given in the written form.

- ❖ Medication cards can be a helpful aid
- ❖ Patient information leaflets (PILs)

Patient Counselling and Medication Adherence

Drug attendance is the degree to which a person follows medical guidance when taking their medications. The following outcomes could occur if people disregard their doctor's instructions:

- Failure of treatment,
- An increased risk of hospitalization,
- Increased medical and non-medical costs, and
- Lower quality of life

Informing patients about their medications helps them follow instructions and avoid these issues.

Qualities of a good counsellor

Be a good listener: Counselling is an interactive process, so listen well. Pharmacists must watch and attend to patients. The chemist can gauge the patient's illness and drug expertise.

Be flexible: The chemist should adapt the advice to the patient's wants and skills.

Be empathetic: The chemist should feel the patient's pain as if it were theirs.

Be non-judgmental: The pharmacy should not rate patients' behaviour based on their disease or group.

Be tolerant: Counseling patients may become anxious, irrational, or angry. Pharmacists should respect patients' emotions.

Be Confident: Confidence will help patients take the pharmacist's advice.

Some Important Aspects of Counselling

1. **Environment:** Patient-pharmacist contact should be easy. Privacy and time for contact are needed.
2. **Benefits:** Information benefits people greatly. Pharmacies gain revenue.
3. **Barriers**

Barriers are three types

- ✓ **Patient-Based Barriers:** Patients may not listen. He/she may be disabled, shy, or illiterate. Patience is needed to surmount these hurdles, but if the patient refuses to advise, leave him alone.
- ✓ **System-based Barriers:** The establishment's owners may dislike or lack room for patient therapy.
- ✓ **Provider-Based Barriers:** The pharmacy advice may have language, topic, or other issues. To properly advise patients, these obstacles must be defeated.

Recent Developments

Despite the difficulties stated above, some neighbourhood pharmacists are interested in teaching their customers how to use medications.

Additionally, they provide various health monitoring services, including blood pressure and blood sugar testing.

State pharmacy organizations offer ongoing education courses to help working pharmacists stay current in understanding medicines and counselling techniques.

Documentation

Pharmacists' registers

Pharmacists should keep a highly confidential record that includes the following information:

- patient information,
- disease counselled,
- date and time, and
- patient comments and follow-up.

Effective patient counselling aims to produce the following results:

- A better comprehension of the patient's disease and the function of medicine in its management.
- Increased devotion to medicine.
- More efficient medication therapy.
- A decrease in drug mistakes, side effects, and needless medical expenses.
- Patient's quality of life was improved.
- More effective coping mechanisms for side effects brought on by medicine.
- A stronger working relationship between the pharmacy and the customer.

Study questions:

1. Enumerate the barriers to effective patient counselling.
2. Importance of patient counselling.
3. Enlist the qualities of a patient counsellor.
4. Write the various patient counselling aids.
5. Mention the benefits of professional relationships with other healthcare professionals.
6. Preparation of written and verbal drug information query reports and documentation.
7. Discuss patient counselling technique.
8. Examples of open-ended and closed-ended question.

PATIENT COUNSELLING FORM

I.P.NO   Date:
Code No:
Age: Sex:
Wt:

Past Medical History:

Family Medical History:
Social History:

Past Medication History:

Current Illness:

Allergies (drug/food/other):

Current Medication:

Counseling given on:

Patient perception with respect to disease and medication:

Patient compliance and evaluation:

Poor ☐   Satisfactory ☐   Good ☐

Major side effects and management:

Counseling Points:

A. Precautions:

Clinical Pharmacy: A Practical Manual

B. Diet and exercise:

C. Interactions (drug-drug, drug-food, drug-disease):

D. Storage:

Information on missed doses:

Any communication barriers:

Yes ☐   No ☐

If Yes:

Language ☐   Literacy ☐   Physical (sensory impairment)

Anxiety ☐   Age ☐   Time ☐   Non- co operative

How was the barrier overcome?

Name of Patient: Sign:

Name of Pharmacist: Sign:

Name of Faculty-Incharge: Sign:

Experiment No: 3

INTERPRETATIONS OF LABORATORY INVESTIGATIONS

AIM: To Interpret the Laboratory Investigations

BLOOD CHEMISTRY TESTS

1. Blood studies, called "blood chemistry tests," quantify the levels of specific compounds in a blood sample.
2. They can help detect anomalies and demonstrate how well specific systems are functioning.
3. Chemistry panels are another name for blood chemistry exams.
4. Blood chemical exams come in a variety of forms.
5. In addition to enzymes, ions, fats (also known as lipids), hormones, carbohydrates, proteins, vitamins, and minerals are among the substances they assess.
6. Frequently, multiple compounds are combined and analyzed simultaneously.

Reason for conducting blood chemistry tests

Blood studies that measure blood composition are frequent. An abnormally high or low chemical level in the blood may indicate illness in the organ or tissue that produces it. Although they can be done at any moment, they are frequently performed as part of a regular checkup.

Blood chemistry tests can be done to:

- Acquire knowledge about overall health.
- Examine the functionality of specific organs, such as the thyroid, liver, and kidneys.
- Verify the chemical equilibrium in the body.
- Assist with illness and condition diagnosis.
- Give the chemical concentrations (a benchmark) for comparison with upcoming blood chemistry studies.

Interpretations of Laboratory Investigations

- ➤ Monitor the impact of therapy on specific systems.
- ➤ Keep an eye on cancer or other conditions (as a part of follow-up).

Common blood chemistry tests

Different tests may be used to measure different types of chemicals. The following are some standard blood chemistry tests.

BASIC METABOLIC PANEL (BMP)

A collection of essays known as the basic metabolic panel (BMP) examines several compounds in the blood. One of the most frequently requested laboratory procedures is it. The BMP provides the medical professional with crucial details regarding the body's metabolism (hence the metabolic panel). The BMP offers data on the amount of blood sugar (glucose), the pH and fluid equilibrium, and renal health. An issue that needs to be handled and may call for additional testing can be indicated by anomalous findings, particularly combos of abnormal results.

The BMP includes the following tests:

A. BLOOD GLUCOSE LEVEL:

- The only energy source for the brain and nerve system, glucose serves as the body's main fuel supply.
- Both a stable quantity and a broadly consistent blood glucose level must be kept accessible for use.
- This examination is used to detect diabetes and prediabetes and to check for excessive blood sugar (hyperglycemia) or insufficient blood sugar (hypoglycemia).
- The usual range for fasting blood sugar is 60 to 100 mg/100 millilitres.
- After taking 50 milligrams of glucose, the blood sample is removed after two hours.

- Within one to two hours, blood sugar levels revert to normal after reaching a peak.
- It suggests diabetes mellitus if the amount does not drop and stays high for more than 50 milligrams above the fasting value.
- Elevated blood sugar is a sign of hyperthyroidism, liver problems, pancreas illness, and hyperglycemia.
- Insufficient blood sugar levels are seen in conditions like hyperthyroidism, hypopituitarism, and insulin overdose.

B. BLOOD CALCIUM LEVEL:

- The most prevalent and one of the most vital elements in the body, calcium is crucial for healthy cell signalling and the smooth operation of the heart, muscles, and neurons.
- Calcium is essential for bone and tooth development, blood coagulation and bone and tooth care.
- This examination examines the calcium levels in the blood or urine, which reflect the body's total and ionic calcium levels.
- There are two procedures to assess blood calcium levels.
- The total calcium assay measures both unbound and bonded types of calcium.
- Only the liberated, biologically active type of calcium is measured by the ionized calcium test.
- Adult blood calcium levels should be within the standard range of 8.6–10.2 mg/dL.
- There is no set standard limit for children, however.
- Conditions like hyperparathyroidism, malignant cells, hyperthyroidism, sarcoidosis, TB, etc., may cause higher total calcium levels (hypercalcemia) than the standard number.
- However, liver illness or starvation, hypoparathyroidism, reduced levels of vitamin D, magnesium insufficiency, elevated levels of phosphorous, severe gastritis, kidney failure, etc., may be the causes of lower total calcium levels (hypocalcemia).

AN ELECTROLYTE PANEL

It helps identify bodily fluid and chemical imbalance issues. The major ions in the body are measured by the electrolyte panel, including:

- Sodium
- Potassium
- Chloride
- Magnesium
- Phosphate
- Bicarbonate

Sodium:
- All bodily secretions contain sodium, essential for maintaining regular bodily functions like neuron and muscular activity.
- This examination determines the blood's salt content.
- An aberrant sodium amount, such as insufficient sodium (hyponatremia) or excessive sodium is detected by a sodium blood test (hypernatremia).
- The standard sodium range for adults is 136-145 mmol/L, but for people over 90 years old, it is 132-146 mmol/L.
- Diarrhea, vomiting, excessive perspiration, the use of medications, renal disease, low levels of cortisol, aldosterone, and sex hormones (Addison disease), swelling brought on by heart failure, etc., are among the conditions that can result in reduced blood sodium (hyponatremia). Dehydration, Cushing syndrome, diabetes insipidus, and other conditions can result in hypernatremia, a disease where blood sodium levels are elevated.

Potassium
- For cells to function correctly, potassium, an element, must help carry nutrition into the cells and eliminate waste products from them.

- It aids in communicating signals between neurons and muscles, which is crucial for proper muscular performance.
- This test is used to determine the level of potassium in the blood. It is carried out whenever a chemical imbalance is thought to cause symptoms like muscle fatigue and/or erratic heartbeat (cardiac arrhythmia).
- Adult blood potassium levels should be within the standard 3.5-5.1 mmol/L range.
- Kidney illness, exhaustion, diabetes, addison disease, tissue damage, and medications like non-steroidal anti-inflammatory medicines (NSAIDs), ACE inhibitors, and beta blockers are among the conditions that can result in elevated potassium levels (hyperkalemia).
- However, gastrointestinal disorders like diarrhea and vomiting, primary hyperaldosteronism (Conn syndrome), acetaminophen overdose complications, diabetes, and specific medications like corticosteroids and beta-adrenergic agonists are some of the conditions that can result in lower potassium levels (hypokalemia).

Chloride

- It is a negatively charged particle that collaborates with other ions to stabilize the body's acid-base equilibrium, including potassium, sodium, and bicarbonate.
- This procedure evaluates the blood's chlorine content.
- While chloride can be found in all bodily fluids, it is most abundant in blood and extracellular fluid surrounding the body's cells.
- Most of the time, chloride concentrations rise and fall for the exact causes and in direct proportion to sodium, just like sodium concentrations do.
- However, because chloride serves as a cushion when there is an acid-base mismatch, blood chloride levels can alter without regard to sodium levels.

Interpretations of Laboratory Investigations

- By migrating into or out of the cells as necessary, it aids in maintaining electrical balance at the cellular level.
- Adult blood Cl- levels should be within the standard range of 98–107 mmol/L.
- Chloride levels can be low or elevated due to several ailments and illnesses.
- While an elevated blood chloride level (also known as hyperchloremia) typically suggests exhaustion, it can also be a symptom of other conditions that raise blood sodium levels, such as Cushing syndrome or renal illness.
- Hyperventilation or excessive base loss from the body, which results in metabolic acidity, may also cause increased blood chloride levels (causing respiratory alkalosis).
- Any condition that lowers blood sodium can also cause a drop in blood chloride or hypochloremia.
- Insufficient chloride can also be a symptom of pulmonary acidosis, congestive heart failure, diabetic ketoacidosis, aldosterone insufficiency, extended regurgitation, stomach aspiration, Addison disease, emphysema, or other persistent lung illnesses, as well as when the body stops producing acid (called metabolic alkalosis).

Bicarbonate

- The body uses bicarbonate, a chemical and negatively charged particle, to help keep its acid-base (pH) equilibrium.
- In order to keep the electrical balance at the cellular level, it also collaborates with the other ions (sodium, potassium, and chloride).
- This examination examines the overall concentration of blood carbon dioxide (CO_2), primarily bicarbonate (HCO_3^-).
- The majority of CO_2 is a byproduct of different biological activities.

- Adult blood bicarbonate (HCO3-) levels should be within the standard range of 23 to 29 mmol/L. Addison disease, persistent dysentery, diabetic ketoacidosis, metabolic acidosis, and pulmonary alkalosis, which can be brought on by hyperventilation shock, renal disease, etc., are all conditions that can result in low bicarbonate levels.
- Conditions resulting in a high bicarbonate level include metabolic alkalosis, lung illnesses like COPD, severe and protracted sickness and/or diarrhea, and lung diseases like Cushing syndrome and Conn syndrome.

KIDNEY FUNCTION TEST/ RENAL PANEL

Blood urea nitrogen (BUN):

- Urine is a waste product that the kidneys remove from circulation.
- BUN content increases as kidney efficiency declines.
- This test is used to assess the condition of the kidneys, aid in diagnosing renal disease, and track the efficacy of dialysis and other therapies for kidney injury or disease.
- Blood urea nitrogen standard limits for adults and people over 60 are 2.1–7.1 mmol/L and 2.9–8.2 mmol/L, respectively.
- Kidney illness, exhaustion, consuming more protein, chronic heart failure, shock, tension, recent heart attack, or severe burns are among the circumstances that can cause a rise in BUN values.
- However, liver illness and starvation are the causes of the decline in BUN values.

Serum Creatinine:

- The kidneys remove creatinine, a waste product created in the muscles due to the decomposition of the substance creatine, from the blood.

- This examination aims to determine how well the kidneys are functioning.
- Creatinine test findings are evaluated with BUN test results and any other tests that may have been run concurrently, such as a kidney panel.
- The standard ranges for men and women aged 18 to 60 years are 80 to 115 mol/L and 53 to 97 mol/L, respectively.
- However, the male and female >60 yr age groups have 71 - 115 mol/L and 53 - 106 mol/L, respectively.
- Higher serum creatinine levels can be caused by glomerulonephritis, pyelonephritis, shock, dehydration, congestive heart failure, atherosclerosis, or diabetic complications, as well as conditions that reduce blood flow to the kidney.
- Low blood creatinine levels are uncommon and typically not a cause for concern.

Blood Cholesterol

In healthy young people, the normal range is between 100 and 240 mg/100 mL, steadily increasing with age. A severe sign of heart disease in young people is an elevated blood cholesterol level of 300 mg/100 mL.

Significance:

- A rise in blood cholesterol is linked to several clinical illnesses, including nephrosis, lipemia, diabetes mellitus, hypothyroidism, and hepatitis.
- Blood cholesterol declines are brought on by hyperthyroidism, pernicious anemia, wasting disease, severe illnesses, and liver damage.

HAEMATOLOGICAL PARAMETERS

❖ **Erythrocytes (Red Blood Cells):**

The total RBC count of blood is expressed as the number of cells per mm.

Significance:

- A rise in circulating RBCs, either relative or absolute, is a pathological situation that causes polycythemia (erythrocytosis) and is seen in many different pathological conditions like persistent heart disease, dysentery, and burns.
- Pregnancy, anemia, etc., are conditions where a drop in RBC counts is seen.

❖ **Leucocytes (White blood cells):**

The total leucocyte count is expressed as the number of WBC in cubic mm of whole blood.

Significance:

- The presence of an illness, such as a viral infection, fever, sinusitis, diphtheria, measles, or cold, is indicated by an increase in WBCs.
- Increased WBC counts indicate physiological leucocytosis in pregnancy, newborns, hormonal disorders, menstruation, anxiety, and other conditions.
- Significant growth indicates leukemia.

WBC differential analysis gives the distribution of various types of leucocytes.

❖ **Basophils:**
- Numerous clinical diseases, including granulocytic leukemia, lymphocytic leukemia, breast cancer, viral hepatitis, mumps, varicella, and viral hepatitis, all show a rise in basophil numbers.

- ❖ **Eosinophils**:
  - An increase in eosinophils, or eosinophilia, is a sign of allergic conditions like bronchial asthma, eczema, and food allergies, as well as skin conditions like pruritus, leprosy, and exfoliative dermatitis, as well as diseases like cholera, scarlet fever, ovarian and uterine tumours, ulcerative colitis, and others.
  - Stress, Cushing disease, and acute illnesses are associated with decreased eosinophils.
- ❖ **Monocytes:**
  - These cells are phagocytic.
  - Malaria, ulcerative colitis, monocytic leukemia, TB, and other bacterial diseases are all known to cause a noticeable rise in monocytes (monocytosis).
- ❖ **Lymphocytes:**
  - Children with viral infections (measles, mumps, whooping cough) and lymphocytosis (lymphocyte increase) are affected.
  - Other dangerous diseases include breast cancer, gonorrhea, and TB.
  - A decrease in lymphocytes, or lymphocytopenia, can indicate Hodgkin's disease, heart failure, stress, the AIDS virus, end-stage kidney failure, etc.
- ❖ **Neutrophils:**
  - Neutrophils leukocytosis (an increase in neutrophils) is seen in conditions such as necrosis, cardiac infarction, rheumatic fever, and rheumatoid arthritis.
  - Malaria, dengue, infective hepatitis, TB, typhoid, paratyphoid, etc., cause neutropenia (a drop in neutrophils).
- ❖ **Thrombocytes (Platelets):**

The cores of platelets are very tiny, measuring only 3. They are essential for the clotting of blood.

    Significance:

- Thrombocytosis (an increase in the number of thrombocytes) is seen in several illnesses, including Hodgkin's disease, cirrhosis of the liver, severe hemorrhage, and TB.
- Thrombocytopenia (reduction in platelet count) is a sign of myeloproliferative diseases, major hemorrhage, Gaucher's disease, septicemia, splenic hypertrophy, and other conditions like miliary TB.

❖ **Haemoglobin:**
- Haemoglobin indicates red blood cells' ability to transport oxygen.
- Anaemia is a disease marked by insufficient hemoglobin levels.
- Their levels of polycythemia and exhaustion are above average.

❖ **ESR. or Erythrocyte Sedimentation Rate:**
- In this method, whole blood's erythrocytes (RBCs) can gravitationally settle over time (usually 1 hr).
- The sedimentation rate, expressed in millimetres per hour, is the rate at which they fall. To identify tissue injury in a variety of diseases, such as cardiac ischemia and angina pectoris, ESR. is very helpful.
- Myocardial infarction, rheumatoid arthritis, rheumatic fever, tuberculosis, kidney illness, cancer, anemia, pneumonia, measurement, etc., are all associated with rising ESR.
- Sickle cell anemia, polycythemia vera, and other conditions indicate a fall in ESR.

❖ **The clotting time of blood:**
- It is the amount of time needed for blood to coagulate, at which point fibrinogen is changed into fibrin to create a framework for fixing the cellular component.

Interpretations of Laboratory Investigations

- At 370C, the standard limit for whole-body coagulation duration is 4 to 9 minutes.

Significance:

- It is used to identify conditions like leukemia, blocked hepatitis, vitamin K shortage anemia, and hemophilia.
- A lengthy bleeding period indicates hemophilia (factor VIII deficiency).
- Clotting time is typically monitored before surgery to limit excessive blood loss.

URINE EXAMINATION

- When there is a sick state of the body, abnormal components appear in the urine sample.
- Urine is typically analyzed chemically, physiologically, and microscopically.
- Numerous bodily examinations, including those for volume, look, pH, and specific gravity, are carried out to gather fundamental data on several systemic illnesses.

GENERAL STOOL EXAMINATION

❖ **Macroscopic observation of the fecal sample:**
  1. The types of microbes can be inferred from the stool's macroscopic look. Normal feces have a consistent shape. The feces are semi-solid or liquid in cases of diarrhea and dysentery. Most cysts have been discovered in solid feces, whereas trophozoites have predominately been discovered in liquid stools.
  2. Colour: Bile compounds make adult stools ordinarily dark, and the type of food consumed impacts stool colour. Yellow-green and semi-formed infant excrement are typical.

❖ **Abnormal types of feces colour:**

1. Watery (like rice water): The cholera sufferer was watery (like rice water) (Vibrio cholerae)

2. Clay or white coloured: Blocked jaundice or the colour of clay, or the presence of barium sulphate

3. Reddish coloured: Blood from the lower GI system and meat intake are reddish.

4. Black: Charcoal, iron, and upper gastric bleeding (melena).

5. Green: Consuming spinach and taking antibiotics.

The appearance of sputum, blood, or mucous

The presence of adult worms can also be seen in freshly passed stool eggs in the adult stages of Ascaris lumbricoides and Enterobius vermicularis. Proglottid of Taenia species can also be seen.

Blood and mucus: Entameoba histolytica is the source of amoebic diarrhea.

The diagnosis is blood and pus: Shigella, Compylobacter, or E. Coli-caused bacillary dysentery.

Only Blood: If there is only blood, Salmonella, E. Coli, or Clostridium difficile-caused diarrhea is the diagnosis.

❖ **Microscopic examination**

Examine fecal specimens under (10X and 40X objectives) of a light microscope and report the presence of:

- A large number of pus cells.
- Shigellosis is characterized by clumps of pus cells with > 50 cells per high power field, macrophages, and erythrocytes.
- Cholera, EPEC, ETEC, and viral diarrhea all have fewer pus cells than other types of diarrhea, with fewer than 5 cells per high power field.
- RBCs.

- Flagellates, eggs, embryos, tumours, amoebas.

❖ **Chemical Examination of Stool**
- pH: Normally, stools have a neutral pH. (pH 6).
- In bacillary dysentery, the pH of the feces is alkaline, whereas it is acidic in amoebic dysentery.
- Occult blood: Occult blood may be found in various illnesses, such as GI tract cancer (colon, rectum, stomach).
- Reducing factors: mono- and di-sugar levels in stools (6 mg/g), any rise indicating an imbalance in the enzymes responsible for digesting sugar (e.g., Lactase, Sucrase).

EXAMINATION FOR COMMON ENZYMES

❖ **Phosphatases:**
- These enzymes facilitate the separation of mono-phosphoric acid esters from phosphoric acid.
- The serum contains two different kinds of phosphatases.
- Acid phosphatase is most active around pH 5, and alkaline phosphatases are most active around pH 10.
- Serum acid phosphatase levels should be between 1 and 5 KA units/100 millilitres.
- Prostatic cancer enhances its occurrence.
- Alkaline phosphatase levels should be between 29 and 92 IU/L in the blood. Higher amounts are seen in rickets, osteomalacia, poor vitamin D uptake, calcium deficiency, and diarrhea.

❖ **Serum Glutamate Oxaloacetate Transaminase (SGOT):**
- Up to 35 SF units/100 millilitres is the average concentration of this enzyme. Infective, toxic hepatitis, cirrhosis, blocked jaundice, heart conditions (myocardial ischemia), and muscular injury cause a rise in SGOT values.

❖ **Serum Glutamate Pyruvate Transaminase (SGPT) or Alanine Transaminase (ALT):**
- At 37°C, it catalyzes the conversion of L-alanine to pyruvate.

- The typical SGPT limit is 35 SF units/100 mL. (sigmafrankel units). Damage to liver cells is at an elevated degree.

❖ **Diastase in Urine:**
- Starch is affected by the diastase enzyme in pee, which turns it into maltose.
- Urine diastase should be within the range of 3-32 units. Pancreatitis causes a rise in urinary diastase activity.

❖ **Lactic Acid Dehydrogenase (LHD or LD):**

This enzyme catalyzes the interconversion of lactate and pyruvate. There are 5 LHD isoenzymes, and they are each characterized as follows:

- LHD1 and LHD2 present in the heart
- LHD3 in the lungs
- LHD4 and LHD5 mainly in liver and skeletal muscle
- Their distribution aids in diagnosing numerous clinical conditions, including liver and cardiac ischemia.

❖ **Creatine Phosphokinase (CPK):**
- Both skeletal muscle and cardiac tissue contain it.
- CPK has three isoenzymes: CPK-MH (for the muscle), CPK-BB (for the brain), and CPK-MB. (Heart).
- Differentiate the harm caused by measuring their degree.

Study Questions:

1. Write the Cockcroft-Gault Equation
2. Explain the different hematological tests useful in classifying types of anemias and the standard values.
3. Discuss the importance of various thyroid function tests
4. Discuss in brief Cardiac Markers
5. Explain the different methods of microbial culture sensitivity tests
6. Clinical Implications of commonly ordered Renal Function Tests.
7. Name the 2 drugs altering serum Sodium levels
8. Write the significance of ESR values
9. Significance of the presence of protein and glucose in the urine

Clinical Pharmacy: A Practical Manual

LABORATORY INTERPRETATION FORM

Case No:

IP/OP No:	DOA: __/__/____ DOD: __/__/____		Consultant:
Patient Name:	Bed No:	Time:	Department/Unit:
Age: Sex:	Ht (inches): Wt (Kgs): BMI:		Shift: Morning/Afternoon
Chief Complaints on Admission:			
Present Medical & Medication History:			
Past Medical History:	Past Medication History:		
Social History: Smoking: Yes/No; if yes _/day Alcohol: Yes/No; if yes _____ Quantity Chewing tobacco: Yes/No; if yes _____ Quantity	Allergies: Food: (Veg/Non-Veg) Drug: Others:		
	Pregnancy Status (if applicable):		
Family History:	Surgical History:		

Interpretations of Laboratory Investigations

Physical Examination		Systemic Examination
Vital Signs/Date	CVS:	
Blood pressure (mmHg):	RS:	
Pulse Rate (/min):	Abdomen:	
Respiratory rate (/min):	GIT:	
Temperature (^{0}F):	GU:	
Heart rate (bpm):	CNS:	
SpO2	Clubbing:	
pH:	Anemic:	
Others	Pallor:	
	Oedema:	
	Pupil:	

Provisional Diagnosis:

Lab Investigations		
Biochemical Report	**Complete Blood Picture**	**Complete Urine Examination**
FBS: 60-110mg/dl	Hb: 11-16.5 g/dL-F 14.3-18 g/dL -M	Colour
PBS: Upto 140mg/dl	PCV: 35-50 g%	Appearance
RBS: <160mg/dl	RBC: 3.8-4.8ml/ m^3- F 4.5-6.5ml/m^3 -M	Reaction
Hb1AC: 4.7-6.4%	WBC: 4000-11000 cells/m^3	Specific Gravity
Sodium: 135-146meq/l	Platelet: 1.5-4.0 Lac/m^3	Protein
Potassium: 3.5-5.1meq/l	Neutrophils: 40-75%	Sugar
Chloride: 95-105meq/l	Lymphocytes: 20-40%	Ketone bodies
Calcium: 8.4-10.2mg/dl	Monocytes: 2-10%	Bile salts
Blood Urea: 10-50 mg/dl	Eosinophils: 1-6%	Bile pigments
Uric Acid: 2.4 - 7.0 mg/dL	Basophils: 0-1%	Urobilinogen
Se. Creatinine: 0.5-1.5 mg/dl	ESR: <20mm 1st Hr	Blood
	MCV: 80-100Fl	Epithelial cells

Clinical Pharmacy: A Practical Manual

	MCH: 26.5-33.5		Pus cells	
	MCHC: 31.5-35.0		RBC	
			Casts	
			Crystals	
Liver Function Tests Parameters	**Lipid Function Tests**		**Thyroid Function Tests**	
Parameters	**Parameters**		**Parameters**	
Tot. bilirubin: 0.22-1.0mg/dl	Cholesterol: <200mg/dl		T3: 0.8-2.0ng/ml	
Direct bilirubin: 0-02mg/dl	HDL: >50mg/dl		T4: 5.13-14.06ug/dl	
Indirect bilirubin: T.B-D.B	LDL: <100mg/dl		TSH: 0.46-4.7Iu/ml	
SGPT(ALT): Upto 45U/L	Triglycerides: <150 mg/dl			
SGOT(AST): 5-40U/L	**Other Parameters**		**Other Tests**	
Tot. protein: 5.5-8.0gm/dl				
Albumin: 3.5-5.0gm/dl				
Globulin: 2.0-3.5gm/dl				
A/G ratio:				
A/G ratio:				

Culture and Sensitivity: | **U/S:**

X-Ray / CT scan / MRI: | **ECG / 2D ECHO:**

Other Notes:

Assessment:

Final Diagnosis:

Experiment No: 4

PATIENT MEDICATION HISTORY INTERVIEW

AIM: To interview regards the patient's medication history:

INTRODUCTION:

Medical history is a thorough, accurate, and comprehensive account of every prescription and over-the-counter drug a patient has ever taken or is taking before beginning new inpatient or outpatient treatment. It offers insightful information about a patient's allergy propensity, compliance with pharmaceutical and non-pharmacological therapies, drug use in social situations, and potential use of complementary and traditional medications for self-medication. Medication history interviews are conducted when gathering information about a patient's medical background.

The patient's drug background offers essential insights into the patient's propensity for allergies, compliance, and self-medication. A pharmacy can create a pharmacological care plan and build a relationship with a patient through this practice.

OBJECTIVE:

A medical history discussion aims to gather details about drug use that may help with the patient's general treatment.

The information gathered can be utilized to:

- ➤ Investigate any inconsistencies by comparing drug characteristics and medicine delivery records.
- ➤ Verify the drug histories of other staff members and offer more details as needed.
- ➤ Record sensitivities and negative responses.
- ➤ Check for possible medication problems.
- ➤ Evaluate the patient's adherence to medicine.
- ➤ Evaluate the justification for the medication recommended.

- Analyze the substance misuse proof.
- Evaluate the methods used to administer medications.
- Examine whether any medical assistance is required.
- Record medicine delivery requested by the patient.

Importance of Accurate Medication History:

- Assists in preventing medication mistakes and the associated dangers to patients.
- Helpful in identifying drug-related diseases and any clinical symptoms brought on by the effects of drug treatment.
- An improved patient treatment plan can be created by considering all the correct details about their drug background.

PROCEDURE:

Stages of Patient Medication History

The patient drug history practice process involves three steps.

Below is a discussion of each stage's goal and process:

- ❖ **Stage 1: Before taking medication, history.**
  Objective: To establish trust with people and foster positive interactions.
  Method: Following are different steps in this procedure:
  - Verifying the patient's name.
  - Self-Introduction.
  - The purpose of the questioning and the length of time needed.
  - Begin gathering a patient's drug information.

- ❖ **Stage 2: During the taking of history.**
  Objective: To collect accurate information on the medication history.

Method:
Ask the query in the manner prescribed for the gathering of medication-related data.

❖ **Stage 3: After taking history.**
   Objective: Documentation and analysis of information.
❖ **Method:**
   - The pharmacist must thank the patient for sharing this information after the discussion.
   - Examine and analyze the prior medical file.
   - Recording a patient's critical medical background information.

A Pattern of Questions to Be Asked by Pharmacists in Interview

The inquiries that a pharmacy might ask to gather information about a patient's drug background are listed below.

➢ Which medicines have you taken or are you taking right now?
➢ The brand name of the drug taken.
➢ Dosage form type.
➢ Medication dose.
➢ How (by what path) are they travelling there?
➢ How many times should I consume a day?
➢ What is the purpose of your drug use?
➢ Have adverse responses to medicines been reported, and what was the reaction?
➢ Do you regularly or, as required, take any medications? When you say sure, why?
➢ Are there any over-the-counter drugs that you regularly or occasionally take? When you say sure, why?
➢ Are there any conventional medications that you regularly or occasionally take? When you say sure, why?
➢ Do you take any vitamins or other supplements? When you say sure, why?
➢ Have you ever tried a new medication?

Patient Medication History Interview

- Has your doctor lately changed your medication's dosage or stopped prescribing it?
- Have you recently reduced your dosages or stopped taking any of your medications?
- Are there any adverse effects from any of the medications?
- Did you cease taking medicines or switch them because of adverse side effects or discomfort?
- Did you ever take a break from taking your medication when you felt better?

Information sources:

- Patient
- Family or Caregiver
- Medication Vials
- Medication List
- Community Pharmacy
- Medication Profiles from other facilities
- DPIN (Drug Programs Information Network)

Type of Information Needs to Be Recorded

In order to gather information about the patient's medications, the following details are frequently noted during the patient interview: Recently prescribed medicines.

- Taking over-the-counter drugs.
- Any current or previous immunizations.
- Any societal behaviour (e.g. Alcohol, smoking).
- Any usage of conventional drugs.
- The use of medication brings on allergies and responses.
- Drugs were discovered to be useless.
- Adherence to prior therapy.
- Making use of any methods or aids for administering or adhering to medicine.

Study Questions:

1. Significance of Medication History interview.
2. Discuss in brief the steps involved in the Medication history interview.
3. Structure of patient case history.

Patient Medication History Interview

MEDICATION HISTORY INTERVIEW FORM

Patient Name:	Gender:	Consultant:
Ward:	Admission Date:	Interview Date:
Email id:	IP No:	Case No:

1. Reminder Preference: I would like to receive preventive and follow-up care reminders.

Yes   No

2. Allergies: Do you have any allergies to drugs/food? If yes, what drug/food and type of allergic reaction?

3. Medical conditions: Do you have any past or present medical conditions? If yes, mention the condition.

4. Diagnostic Tests/Studies: Did you go for any diagnostic studies or test/s earlier? If yes, when and what type of tests were they?

A) Do you have any report of the performed test/s? If yes, please let us see the report/what is the impression of the test report?

8. Surgeries & Procedures: Do you have any previous surgeries or procedures? If yes, mention what it was.

9. Marital Status: What is your marital status? Mention single/married/divorced/separated/ widowed/civil union

10. Family Medical History: Is there any family medical history? If yes, what are the relationship status and their diagnosis?

11. Prescribed Medication: (What medicines are you having at the moment?)

A) Record here what the patient says; note any anomalies with their current prescription.

B) Other drugs prescribed previously (with date if possible): What have you had in the past?

Patient Medication History Interview

12. Non-Prescribed Medication: Do you take anything that you buy from a shop without a prescription chemist, health food stores, and supermarkets?

A) Currently being used

B) Used previously (with dates if possible)

13. Social Drugs: What social habits do you have, and how much/many per week?

A) Smoking:

B) Alcohol:

C) Chewing tobacco:

D) Illicit Drugs:

14. Immunizations: Did you take any vaccinations earlier? If yes, mention when and what type of vaccinations.

15. Response to drug therapy

A) Do you think your current medication is benefitting you?

If yes, how?

If not, why?

B) Do you think your previous medication benefited you?

If yes, which one and how?

If not, why?

---

16. Do any of the things you buy without a prescription help you?

If yes, how and which ones

---

17. Side Effects:

A) Are you suffering any side effects now? If yes, what side effects?

B) Which of your medicines do you think is causing the problems?

Patient Medication History Interview

C) Have you suffered any side effects with previous drug treatments? If yes, what and with which medicines?

18. Compliance:

A) How do you remember to take your medicines?

B) What do you do when you miss a dose?

19. What medicines would you usually take?

A) Headache

B) Aches/Pains and Flu:

C) Allergy

D) Others_____

20. To whom would you ask for medicines for the problem mentioned above

A) Pharmacist/Chemist

B) Relative or friend C) Nurse: D) Doctor: E) No one:	
21. Any other problems with drug therapy?	
22. Comments	
23. Recommendations	
Consent to Import Medication History: I consent to obtain a history of medical and medication history.	|it
Patient Sign:	**Interviewer sign:**

Experiment No: 5

ADVERSE DRUG REACTION DETECTION AND MANAGEMENT

AIM: ADR detection & management

INTRODUCTION:

Adverse drug reaction (ADR):

An adverse drug reaction is an unpleasant and unexpected response that happens when a drug is taken at a dosage typically used in people for the prevention, detection, or treatment of illness or to alter bodily function.

Adverse Events:

Any unfavourable medical incident that may occur while taking medication but does not necessarily have a causal relationship is considered an adverse event.

The difference between an adverse drug reaction and an adverse event is that the former has a possibility of a causative relationship between the medication and the reaction. In contrast, the latter does not always have such a causal relationship.

Pharmacovigilance: According to the WHO, Pharmacovigilance is the science and activities relating to the detection, assessment, understanding and prevention of adverse effects or any other medicine-related problem.

Activities involved in it

- ❖ Post-marketing surveillance
- ❖ Dissemination of ADR data
- ❖ Changes in the labelling of medicines

WHO Programme for International Drug Monitoring:

- The WHO's Programme for International Drug Monitoring was established in 1968 to combine the available ADR statistics.
- The network was initially a trial initiative in ten nations with national reporting systems for ADRs. However, as more nations globally created national Pharmacovigilance centers for tracking ADRs, it considerably grew.
- Currently, many nations participate in the initiative, which the WHO runs and is cooperating center in Uppsala, Sweden. (UMC).
- Vigibase, the worldwide ADR database, is maintained by the cooperating center.
- WHO plays a significant part in providing professional guidance on all issues pertaining to the safety of medications.

The WHO Collaborating Centre analyses the reports in the database to:

- Recognize the early warning signs of severe medication side effects.
- Assess the risk.
- Conduct a study to understand better how drugs work to create safer and more potent medications.

COMMON CAUSES OF ADRS

- Not taking the proper medications at the correct times.
- Overdosing.
- Allergies to the drug's molecular components.
- Mixing booze and prescription medication.
- Using substances or treatments that interact with the medication.
- Using a prescription drug that was intended for someone else.

FACTORS AFFECTING ADVERSE DRUG REACTIONS:

Patient-related factors

- Age
- Sex
- Genetic influences
- Concurrent diseases (renal, liver, cardiac)
- Previous adverse drug reactions
- Compliance with the dosing regimen
- Total number of medications
- Misc. (diet, smoking, environmental exposure)

AGE

- Because their ability to process substances is typically still developing, children are frequently in danger.
- Acetylsalicylic acid (aspirin) may increase the chance of Reye's syndrome in children under 18 if taken while suffering from chickenpox or influenza.

ELDERLY

- ADRs, such as medication combinations, are a frequent reason for hospital admittance in geriatric patients.
- Elderly ADR causes include:
  - Taking several medicines at once
  - Age-related decreased medication ADME action
- Malnutrition and exhaustion, which are frequent in older people, aggravate these conditions.

PREGNANCY

- Sulfonamides → Jaundice and brain damage in the fetus
- Warfarin → congenital disabilities and increased risk of bleeding problems in newborns and mothers

- Lithium → Defects of the heart (Ebstein's Anomaly), lethargy, reduced muscle tone, and under activity of the thyroid gland

BREASTFEEDING

- • Breast milk is a common way for mothers to transmit medications to their babies.
- Amantadine (antiviral)
- Cyclophosphamide (antineoplastic)
- Cocaine (Schedule 2 FDA drug)
- Carisoprodol (skeletal muscle relaxant)

DRUG-RELATED FACTORS

- Dose
- Duration
- Inherent toxicity of the agent
- Pharmacodynamic properties
- Pharmacokinetic Properties

GENETIC BASIS

BASED ON INCIDENCE Classification

- VERY COMMON
- COMMON
- UNCOMMON
- RARE
- VERY RARE

VERY COMMON ADR

- incidence >10% (1 in 10 people).
- Ex- drowsiness associated with carbamazepine.
- COMMON ADR- incidence is 1-10 to 1-100.
- Ex-fluid retention with carbamazepine.

UNCOMMON ADR

- Incidence 0.1-1.0 % (1-1000 to 1-100)
- Ex- diarrhea associated with carbamazepine.

RARE ADR:

- Incidence 0.01-0.1 % (1-10000 To 1-1000)
- Ex- Depression associated with carbamazepine.

VERY RARE:

- Incdence <0.01% (1-10000).
- EX-arrhythmia associated with carbamazepine.

BASED ON SEVERITY / INTENSITY Classification

- ❖ MILD (minor)
- ❖ MODERATE
- ❖ SEVERE (major)

MILD (minor): Does not require any therapy / may not notice.

MODERATE: Changes needed in medication treatment

SEVER (primary): Able to cause organ damage, serious illness, confinement, or impairment (significant, persistent or permanent, congenital anomaly, required intervention to prevent permanent impairment or damage).

TRADITIONALLY Classification

- ❖ TYPE-A (Augmented)
- ❖ TYPE-B (Bizarre)
- ❖ TYPE-C (continuous)
- ❖ TYPE-D (delayed)
- ❖ TYPE-E (End of Dose)
- ❖ TYPE-F (Failure of therapy)

TYPE-A (Augmented)

Most prevalent (up to 70%) - dosage-dependent; intensity rises with quantity. Generally avoidable if modest doses are introduced gradually. Predictable by pharmaceutical processes.

Such include hypotension produced by beta-blockers, hypoglycemia caused by insulin or dietary hypoglycemics, and stomach sores caused by NSAIDs.

TYPE-B (Bizarre)

Mechanisms are uncommon, peculiar, genetically established, unexpected, unknown, dangerous, and potentially deadly, unconnected to dosage.

Such as hepatitis caused by halothane, chloramphenicol-induced aplastic anemia, antipsychotics, and some anesthetics that can induce neuroleptic malignant syndrome.

TYPE-C (continuous)

The effects of continuing substance use can be permanent, unanticipated, random, and irrevocable.

For instance, dementia is carried on by anticholinergic drugs and tardive dyskinesias are caused by antipsychotics.

TYPE-D (delayed)

The delayed incidence of ADRs, even after therapy has ended.

For example, thioridazine-induced ocular opacities or chloroquine-induced ophthalmopathy.

TYPE-E (End of Dose)

The withdrawal symptoms. This usually happens when taking sedative medication.

For example, convulsions during alcohol or benzodiazepine withdrawal, hypertension and agitation in opioid abstainers, and first-dose hypotension brought on by ACE inhibitors or alpha-blockers (Prazosin).

TYPE-F (Failure of therapy)

Results of ineffective therapy (earlier neglected from analysis following WHO criteria).

Such as increased hypertension because of ineffective management.

HOW TO RECOGNIZE ADRS

- Verify that the patient truly takes the prescribed amount of medication.
- Confirm that the potential ADR started after the medication was taken.
- Calculate the duration between the drug's consumption and the event's start.
- Examine the potential ADR following medication discontinuation or dosage reduction and keep track of progress.
- Examine the potential causes. (Other than the drug).
- Consult pertinent books and a knowledgeable practitioner for advice and information.
- File an ADR.

PROCEDURE FOR REPORTING ADRS

Any pharmacovigilance center's first responsibility is to notify of potential adverse drug reactions.

Details required for reporting ADR events.

Elements in ADR reporting	Necessary information
What should be reported	Adverse reactions to the drug, suspected drug details, patient information **Information required for ADR case reporting** ❖ **Patient information-** • Patient identifier • Age at time of event or date of birth • Gender • Weight ❖ **Adverse event or product problem-** • Description of event or problem • Date of event • Date of this report • Relevant tests/laboratory data (if available) • Other relevant patient information/history • Outcomes attributed to an adverse event. ❖ **Suspected medication (s)** ✓ Name (INN and brand name). ✓ Batch number ✓ Dose, frequency & ✓ Expiration date

Adverse Drug Reaction Detection and Management

Elements in ADR reporting	Necessary information
	route used. ✓ Therapy date. ✓ Diagnosis for use. ✓ The event abated after the use stopped. ✓ Or does reduce ✓ Event reappeared after ✓ Reintroduction of the treatment ✓ Concomitant medical products ✓ And therapy dates ❖ **Reporter:** • Name, address, and telephone number • Specialty and occupation
Who can report	Medical practitioners or health care professionals, doctors, nurses, pharmacists, assistants, pharmaceutical technicians, pharmaceutical assistants, clinical officers, and other health care providers.
When can it be reported	Any adverse reactions, if noticed, should be reported as soon as possible.
How to report	Through filled yellow card form
Where can it be reported	A filled ADR form should be submitted to the pharmacovigilance centre.

WHAT HAPPENS TO THE SUBMITTED INFORMATION?

- Information shared via this form is handled in strict confidence.
- The WHO-UMC is utilized by (AMCs) to perform causality analyses.
- The ADR database transmits the reviewed documents to the National Coordinating Center.
- Finally, the National Coordinating Center occasionally assesses the reports before they are read and sent to the WHO Uppsala Monitoring Center's Global Pharmacovigilance Database. (PvPI).
- The information generated from these records helps with the continuing assessment of the benefit-risk balance of medicines.
- The details are given to the PvPI Steering Committee, established by the Ministry of Health and Family Welfare.
- Reviewing the data and recommending any potential solutions is given to the Committee.

TYPES OF REPORTING

- Internal Reporting
- Spontaneous Reporting
- Voluntary Reporting

MONITORING OF ADR

- WHO-UMC
- NARANJO'S CAUSALITY ASSESSMENT
- HARTWIG SACLE- ADR severity assessment scale

METHODS FOR CAUSALITY ASSESSMENT OF ADRS ARE CLASSIFIED INTO THREE GROUPS:

- Expert opinion, medical expertise, or techniques used for worldwide reflection.
- Standardized evaluation techniques or algorithms (with or without rating).
- Probabilistic or Bayesian approaches.

Adverse Drug Reaction Detection and Management

CAUSALITY ASSESSMENT METHODS

Algorithmic: (algorithm - specify how to solve the problem)

- ❖ Series of questions.
- ❖ Answers are weighted.
- ❖ The overall score determines the causality category.
  e.g. Naranjo's scale.

Probalistic: (based on probability)

- ❖ Set of explicitly defined causality categories
  e.g. WHO UMC method

Uses of causality assessment

- ❖ Initial review of the report
- ❖ Signal detection
- ❖ Scientific publications

WHO Causality Assessments Scale

WHO–UMC causality categories

Causality term	Assessment criteria (all points should reasonably comply)
Certain	✓ Event or anomaly in a lab result possibly related to substance use. ✓ Cannot be attributed to an illness or other medications. ✓ A reasonable response to removal (pharmacologically, pathologically). ✓ Pharmacologically or phenomenologically conclusive event (i.e., an objective and specific medical disorder or a recognized pharmacologic phenomenon). ✓ If required, apply a rechallenge.
Probable/ likely	✓ Event or anomaly in a lab result that relates to substance use.

Causality term	Assessment criteria (all points should reasonably comply)
	✓ Unlikely to be a result of an illness or medication. ✓ The clinically logical response to cessation. ✓ Repetition is not necessary.
Possible	✓ Event or anomaly in a lab result that relates to substance use. ✓ An illness or other medications explain them. ✓ Drug discontinuation information may be lacking or unclear.
Unlikely	✓ An event or aberrant lab result with a time to drug consumption that renders a connection unlikely (but not impossible). ✓ Reasonable explanations include illness or other medications.
Conditional/ unclassified	✓ Anomaly in an event or laboratory test. ✓ For an accurate evaluation, more data are required, or additional data are being looked at.
Unassessable/ unclassifiable	✓ A report suggesting an adverse reaction. ✓ It cannot be judged because the information is insufficient or contradictory. ✓ Data cannot be supplemented or verified.

Naranjo's Causality Assessment Scale

Question	Yes	No	Do not know
Are there previous conclusion reports on this reaction?	+1	0	0
Did the adverse event appear after the suspect drug was administered?	+2	−1	0
Did the adverse reaction improve when the drug was discontinued or a specific antagonist was administered?	+1	0	0
Did the AR reappear when the drug was re-administered?	+2	−1	0
Are there alternate causes [other than the drug] that could solely have caused the reaction?	−1	+2	0
Did the reaction reappear when a placebo was given?	−1	+1	0
Was the drug detected in the blood [or other fluids] in a concentration known to be toxic?	+1	0	0
Was the reaction more severe when the dose was increased or less severe when the dose was decreased?	+1	0	0
Did the patient react similarly to the same or similar drugs in previous exposure?	+1	0	0
Did objective evidence confirm the adverse event?	+1	0	0

Scoring for Naranjo algorithm: >9 = definite ADR; 5–8 = probable ADR; 1–4 = possible ADR; 0 = doubtful ADR.

PREVENTION OF ADR

- Avoid all forms of substance abuse.
- Use of the proper medication dose, dosage form, route and frequency.
- Elicit information about past medication responses and take that into account.
- Identify any allergic illnesses and use caution.
- Anticipation by patient monitoring
    Ex- anemia- due to deficiency of G6PD, check the condition.
- Anticipation of dosage reduction
    Ex- impaired renal / liver function – dosage should reduce
- Monitoring the serum levels(drug)
    Ex- theophylline, aminoglycosides
- Monitoring of pharmacological activity.
    Ex-diuretics- to promote salt & water loss but causes electrolyte depletion & dehydration. So the therapeutic endpoint is not exceeded.
- Can be done by careful observation/monitoring of the patient.
    Ex- patient with meningitis – should be on penicillin.
    Chemotherapy – nausea
- Rule out any potential medication interactions.
- Use the proper medication administration technique.
- Conduct the necessary experimental research.
- Remember that certain meals, booze, and typical home substances can combine.

MANAGEMENT OF ADR

Discontinue the offending agent if -

- It can be halted securely.
- The event is dangerous or unbearable.
- There is a logical alternative.
- The patient's state will get worse if the medicine is kept up.

Continue the medication (modified as needed) if,

Adverse Drug Reaction Detection and Management

- ❖ It is required medically.
- ❖ There is no logical substitute.
- ❖ The issue is minor and will go away over time.
- ❖ Stop taking any unnecessary medicines.
- ❖ Give the proper medical care, such as atropine, protamine sulphate, digibind antibodies, and flumazenil.

Provide supportive or palliative care,

- ❖ Water, glucocorticoids, hot or cold clothes, painkillers, or antipruritics are a few examples.
- ❖ Think about rechallenging or desensitizing.

ROLES OF PHARMACISTS IN THE MANAGEMENT OF ADRs

- Keeping an eye on individuals who are more likely to experience ADRs.
- Keep an eye on patients given medications with a high risk of adverse drug reactions.
- Determining the patient's prior allergy condition and recording it.
- Evaluating the suitability of the patient's medication treatment.
- Examining potential medication combinations across various treatments.
- Assisting healthcare workers in the identification and evaluation of ADRs.
- Stimulating or encouraging medical personnel to report an ADR.
- Recording of alleged reported responses for future use.
- The patient follow-up to evaluate how the response and treatment worked out.
- Getting comments on the supposed response.
- Teaching medical personnel the significance of reporting an ADR.
- Patient education.
- Raising knowledge of ADRs among patients, healthcare providers, and the general public.

- Creation and application of marketing collateral.
- Interaction with other medical specialists, including nurses and neighbourhood pharmacies.
- Reports being presented at seminars and gatherings.
- Holding lectures, symposia, and training on ADRs for medical practitioners.
- The dissemination of signs produced by publishing findings in periodicals or newsletters.

Study Questions:

1. How a pharmacist can involve in the Prevention of ADRs
2. Define ADR. Discuss WHO and Naranjo's scale.
3. Write the pharmacist's role in preventing, monitoring and managing ADRs.
4. Discuss in detail on voluntary reporting of ADRs. Give the reasons for ADRs under-report.
5. Discuss the predisposing factors for ADRs.
6. Define and write the importance of Causality Assessment. Explain the WHO scale.
7. Write in brief on the scope and aims of pharmacovigilance. Discuss voluntary.
8. ADR reporting systems in various countries

SUSPECTED ADVERSE DRUG REACTION REPORTING FORM

A. Patient Information

1. Patient Initials _____   2. Age at the time of the event or
3. Date of Birth _____   4. Sex _____
5. Weight in Kgs: ____

B. Suspected Adverse Reaction

1. Date of Reaction Started:
2. Date of Recovery:
3. Describe the reaction or problem:

C. Suspected Medication(s)

S. No	1. Name (Brand/ Generic)	Manufacturer (if known)	Batch No	Exp. Date	Dose used	Route used	Frequency	Date Started	Date stopped	Reason for Prescribing

S. No.	2. Reaction abated after the drug stopped or the dose reduced					3. Reaction reappeared after reintroduction				
	Yes	No	Unknown	NA	Reduced Dose	Yes	No	Unknown	NA	If reintroduced

4. Concomitant medical products, including self-medication and herbal remedies with therapy dates (exclude those used to treat reactions)

D. Reporter:

Name:
Casualty Assessment:
Date of this report:

Experiment No: 6

MEDICATION ERRORS

AIM: To report Medication Errors

Definition: Medication Error:

The National Coordination Council for Drug Mist Reporting and Prevention defines a drug mistake as follows [NCCMERP].

Any avoidable incident that could result in improper drug use or patient injury while the medication is under the care of the patient, the customer, or the healthcare provider constitutes a medication mistake. These occurrences may have something to do with medical personnel, healthcare goods, practices, and systems, such as prescription writing, order communication, product labelling, selling, dissemination, management, teaching, tracking, and use.

Types of Medication Error

Guidelines provided by the American Society of Hospital Pharmacists (ASHP) classify drug errors into 11 different categories.

1. Prescribing error
2. Omission error
3. Improper dose error
1. Unauthorized drug error
4. Deteriorated drug error
5. Wrong time error
6. Wrong dosage form error
7. Wrong drug preparation error
8. Wrong administration technique error
9. Monitoring error
10. Compliance error

Prescribing Error

- A prescription mistake happens when a doctor prescribes a medication for a particular patient.
- Errors can occur when the wrong amount, dosing type, delivery method, duration of treatment, or several dosages are chosen.
- As an illustration, giving Amoxicillin 250 mg PO TID for a 12-month-old baby would be deemed inappropriate because it would be too high a dosage for a 5-year-old kid with a middle ear infection.

Omission Error

- An absence mistake occurs when a patient is not given a prescribed dosage in a hospital, retirement home, or other institution before the next planned dose.
  -An omission is not a mistake.
  -If there is a health issue.
- Before a treatment, when a patient cannot swallow anything (NPO) or declines to consume them.

Improper Dose Error

- It happens when a patient receives a dosage that is either higher (excess dose error) or lower (underdose error) than what was recommended.
- Causes include failure to record a dosage or a delay in doing so.
- An incorrect dosage mistake can also result from the inaccurate estimation of an ingested beverage.
- The following are excluded from this group:
  - Doses that cannot be accurately measured.
  - Or not specified as in topical application.
  - Metric conversions are excluded as well.

Unauthorized Drug Error

- Giving a patient medicine without the prescribers' appropriate consent is considered an illegal drug mistake.

Medication Errors

- **Causes:**
  1. If a patient's medicine was accidentally provided to another patient.
  2. A nurse administers a drug without a prescription.
  3. Patients who occasionally exchange prescriptions at home.
  4. Refilling a medication without a doctor's permission when no refills are left on it.
  5. Nurses may be incorrect in administering medicine based on patient characteristics.
  6. Dispensing medicine outside of the set parameters.

Deteriorated Drug Error

- Drugs prescribed or given after their expiry date may lose effectiveness or efficacy.
- Refrigerated medications kept at ambient temperature may start to lose their effectiveness.
- Therefore, keeping track of a product's expiry date and storing it properly is crucial.

Wrong Time Errors

- The timing of delivery is essential to a medication's efficacy.
- A sufficient blood volume must be maintained for a medication to be successful.
- Giving dosages too soon or too late may impact the drug's blood level and, as a result, its effectiveness.
- When a patient must leave the patient care area for a test or the medicine is not accessible at that moment, wrong-time mistakes are rarely inevitable.

Wrong Dosage Form Errors

- Mistakes involving dose forms that vary from those prescribed by the physician are called incorrect dosage form mistakes.
- Depending on state legislation and health care centre policies, modifying dose types to meet patient requirements may be permissible.
  - Giving a patient with trouble ingesting pills a liquid version without a prescription might be a suitable dose modification.

Wrong Drug Preparation Error

- Drugs that need reconstitution (adding liquid to a powdery drug), reduction, or other specific processing before being dispensed or administered. However, failure to follow such a process results in incorrect medication production.
    - An erroneous water amount in the sublingual solution of cephalexin is an example. Another example is making a sale with the incorrect essential product.

Wrong Administration Technique Error

- Wrong delivery method mistakes are defined as doses that are given using an unsuitable process or erroneous technique.
    - An overly deep insertion under the skin.
    - An IV medication that does not require an IV machine is administered by gravity.
    - Another illustration is applying ocular medication to the incorrect eye.

Monitoring Errors

- Poor medication treatment evaluation contributes to monitoring mistakes.
    - Prescription of a blood pressure-lowering anti-hypertensive medication without blood pressure check.

Compliance Error

- Patients make medication errors when they don't follow the directions for taking their medications.

Other Error

- The random area is used to combine errors that do not fit into one of the following categories:
    - Calculation error.
    - Decimal points and zero error.
    - Abbreviation error.
    - Look-alike and sound-alike errors.

Medication Errors

Impact of Medication Error:

- Financial problem
- Loss of trust in health care system
- Serious ADR
- Death

Techniques to Prevent the Medication Error:

- Root cause analysis
- Bar check
- Code check
- Colour coding

MEDICATION ERROR REPORTING:

On identifying medication error, the pharmacist reports to the physician

↓

And further, the medication error report form is filled out and forwarded to the MedWatch website.

↓

The reports are being reviewed by the staff of the department DMEPA (a division of medication error prevention and Analysis), which is a part of CDER (center for drug evaluation and Research)

↓

The DMEPA uses the NCCMERP (national coordination council for medication error reporting and Prevention) guidelines to confirm medication errors.

↓

They find the cause and solutions and inform the FDA.

↓

FDA publishes in journals.

Study Questions:

1. Classify Medication Error as per NCC-MERP.
2. Describe the causes of medication errors.
3. Role of pharmacist in the management of Medication error
4. Give 5 examples of look-alike and sound-alike drugs.
5. Classify Medication errors. What are the factors influencing medication errors?
6. Write any five examples of Dispensing errors which you have observed.
7. Write any five examples of Prescribing errors which you have observed.
8. Define Medication errors. Categorize the Medication errors with examples.

Medication Errors

MEDICATION ERROR REPORTING FORM

1. Date of event: _____ Time of event: _____	2. Location of event: _____ ☐ Ward ☐ OPD ☐ Pharmacy ☐ Others_____
3. Type of error: ☐ Prescribing error ☐ Omission ☐ Transcription error ☐ Wrong drug ☐ Dispensing error ☐ Wrong dose ☐ Pharmacy error ☐ Wrong route ☐ Documentation error ☐ Wrong time ☐ Administration error ☐ Refusal ☐ Wrong technique ☐ Others_____	**4. Patient details:** IP No._____ Age: _____ Gender: _____ Diagnosis:_____ **5. Details of the Event:** <table><tr><th>Dosage form</th><th>Generic Name</th><th>Strength</th><th>Frequency</th></tr><tr><td></td><td></td><td></td><td></td></tr><tr><td></td><td></td><td></td><td></td></tr></table>

6. Description of the event (how did the event occur and how it was detected?):

7. Did the error reach the patient? ☐ Yes ☐ No	**8. Outcome of the event:** **No Error** ☐ Events have the potential to cause errors.
9. Possible causes and contributing factors ☐ Lack of knowledge/Experience ☐ Illegible prescription ☐ Look alike/sound like medication. ☐ Wrong labelling/instruction ☐ Use of abbreviations ☐ Unavailable patient information ☐ Peak hour ☐ Miscommunication ☐ Failure to adhere to work procedure	**Error, No harm.** ☐ The error did not reach the patient. ☐ No harm. ☐ No harm, but it requires monitoring. **Error, harm** ☐ Temporary harm requiring treatment. ☐ Temporary harm requiring hospitalization. ☐ Permanent harm ☐ Near-death event **Error, death** ☐ Death

10. Intervention has been done: ☐ Administered antidote   ☐ Changed to correct drug/dose/frequency ☐ No action is needed.   ☐ Education/training provided ☐ Communication process improved ☐ Policy/procedure changed/instituted. ☐ Informed staff who made errors   ☐ Others_____

11. Details of the reporter Name: Designation: Mobile No:	**12. Trainee Pharmacist** Roll No: Name: Sign and date:	**13. Remarks:** Faculty sign and date:

Clinical Pharmacy: A Practical Manual

Experiment No: 7

DRUG UTILIZATION EVALUATION

AIM: To Perform Drug Utilization Evaluation

INTRODUCTION:
- DUE aims to better comprehend drug use and health effects by determining how and why drugs are used the way they are.
- DUE significantly impacts the healthcare system's ability to prescribe, analyze, and enhance the use of medicines.
- DUE data may help institutions and healthcare systems create instructional programs that could enhance medication prescription and usage.
- Some DUE programs might give doctors input on how their performance and prescription habits stack up against preset standards or treatment guidelines.
- Physicians may evaluate their method of managing specific illnesses with that of their colleague's thanks to DUE knowledge.
- These similarities may help encourage doctors to alter their prescription practices to better treatment because they create "peer pressure."
- DUR is still in the process of development.
- Managed care pharmacists can use DUR data to pinpoint prescription patterns in patient demographics and launch remedial action to enhance medication treatment for both groups and people of patients.
- The number of healthcare workers engaged in drug use procedures increases (e.g., pharmacies, prescribers, nurses, optometrists, naturopaths, and chiropractors).
- DUR will necessitate a more interdisciplinary strategy for enhancing patient treatment.
- In addition, the technique for fusing pharmaceutical and medical data with patient result data will be made available by quickly developing data systems.

- This will result in the development of DUR into a more thorough healthcare usage assessment, which is the next natural stage.

Definition:

DUE is a continuous, authorized, and methodical quality development process with the following objectives:

- Review drug use and/or prescription trends.
- Provide doctors and other pertinent groups with input on the findings.
- Establish guidelines and parameters for the best medication use.
- Encourage responsible substance use through initiatives such as instruction.

AIMS OF DUE

The main aim of any DUE study is to promote rational drug use by:

- Reducing the cost of drugs and medical care;
- Enhancing the quality of medical care;
- Enhancing the coordination of healthcare;
- Lowering the incidence of medication-related issues and medication errors;
- Lowering the rate of hospital admissions; and
- Raising prescriber awareness and good prescribing habits.

DRUG UTILIZATION REVIEW

DURs are classified into three categories:

1. Prospective: Assessment of a patient's treatment before administering medicine.

2. Concurrent: Continuous supervision of medication therapy while receiving treatment.

3. Retrospective: An evaluation of the patient's treatment following the administration of the drug.

Prospective DUR:

Before a prescription is filled, a patient's scheduled drug treatment is evaluated as part of a prospective DUR.

This procedure enables the pharmacy to spot potential problems and address them before the patient gets the medicine.

In their regular practice, pharmacists conduct prospective evaluations by examining the dose and instructions for prescribed medications and patient details to check for potential drug conflicts or duplication of treatment.

ISSUES COMMONLY ADDRESSED BY PROSPECTIVE DUR:

- Contraindications for drugs and diseases.
- Therapeutic dialogue.
- Generic replacement.
- Inappropriate medication dose.
- An excessively long course of medication therapy.
- Drug reactions with allergies.
- Clinical negligence or abuse.

Concurrent DUR:

- A concurrent DUR is carried out throughout therapy and entails continuous drug therapy tracking to guarantee successful patient results.
- These days, it is also referred to as case management and health management.
- It allows pharmacists to warn prescribers about possible issues and to step in when necessary in cases like drug-drug combinations, redundant treatment, overuse or underuse, and excessive or inadequate dosage.
- This kind of evaluation enables the patient's treatment to be changed if required. In school environments, concurrent DURs frequently happen.

Drug Utilization Evaluation

ISSUES COMMONLY ADDRESSED BY CONCURRENT DUR:

- Drug-drug interactions.
- Excessive doses.
- High or low dosages.
- Duplicate therapy.
- Drug-disease interactions.
- Over and underutilization.
- Drug-age precautions.
- Drug-gender precautions.
- Drug-pregnancy precautions.

Retrospective DUR:

Retrospective DUR helps prescribers provide better care for their patients, individually and within patient groups, such as those with diabetes, asthma, or high blood pressure, by screening patient medical charts or computerized records to see if the drug therapy met approved criteria.

Issues Commonly Addressed by Retrospective DUR:

- Therapeutic appropriateness.
- Over and underutilization.
- Appropriate generic use.
- Therapeutic duplication.
- Drug-disease contraindications.
- Drug-drug interactions.
- Incorrect drug dosage.
- Inappropriate duration of treatment.
- Clinical abuse/misuse.

Important Of DUR'S

- DUR programs are essential for controlled healthcare systems to comprehend, analyze, and enhance drug prescription, management, and use.

- DUR programs are helpful to employers and health insurers because the outcomes promote more effective use of limited healthcare resources.
- Due to their knowledge of pharmacological treatment, clinical pharmacists play a significant part in this process.
- DURs allow the managed care pharmacy to notice patterns in the prescription of medications for particular patient populations, such as those with chronic illnesses like HIV, cancer, asthma, diabetes, or high blood pressure.
- After that, pharmacists can take action to enhance medication treatment for specific individuals and protected groups, working with other healthcare team members.
- DURs help lower total healthcare costs by enhancing treatment results, increasing patient care quality, and reducing unnecessary medication spending.

The DUE Cycle

It is critical to remember that DUE follows a recurring pattern. The DUE process is ongoing, so completing the cycle instead of carrying out the individual stages separately will be more beneficial.

The DUE cycle should include the following seven significant activities or phases.

1. Planning
2. Data collection
3. Evaluation
4. Feedback of results
5. Interventions
6. Re-evaluation
7. Feedback of results

Drug Utilization Evaluation

Phases and steps involved in conducting a DUE.

Phase I: Planning
Step 1: Identify drugs or therapeutic areas of practice for possible inclusion in the programme
Step 2: Design of the study
Step 3: Define criteria and standards
Step 4: Design the data collection form
Phase II: Data Collection
Step 5: Data collection
Phase III: Evaluation
Step 6: Evaluate the results
Phase IV: Feedback Results
Step 7: Provide feedback on the results
Phase V: Intervention
Step 8: Develop and implement interventions
Phase VI: Re-evaluation
Step 9: Re-evaluate to determine if drug use has improved
Step 10: Re-assess and revise the DUE programme
Phase VII: Feedback Results
Step 11: Feedback results

Possible roles for pharmacists in DUE

- Creating, organizing, and carrying out a DUE schedule.
- The creation, administration, and management of programs.
- Conceptual and actual DUE education for medical personnel.
- Promotion of DUE's aims and purposes.
- The creation and evaluation of audit standards, criteria, research procedures, and instructional materials.
- The creation of data-gathering tools.
- Data gathering, research, and report drafting for pilot testing.
- Documentation of the results, efficiency, and financial advantages of the initiative.

- Participation in medical panels dealing with drug use and quality checking in general.
- Presentation of DUE findings at seminars and gatherings.
- Results publication in peer-reviewed publications.

Study Question:

1. Write on Summary of a due to assess the appropriate ends of ciprofloxacin use.
2. Write the Goals of DUE in the Hospital setup. Explain the Typical DUE cycle in detail.
3. Discuss the protocol and Importance of Drug Utilization Evaluation (DUE).
4. Distinguish DUE & DUR.
5. Differentiate between qualitative and quantitative DUE studies.

www.ingramcontent.com/pod-product-compliance
Lightning Source LLC
Chambersburg PA
CBHW072228170526
45158CB00002BA/796